A Legacy of Hope: The Journey to Cure PSP and Transform Lives

Laura Louizos

DEDICATION

This book is dedicated to my mom, Coleen Cunningham, a PSP warrior who passed in May 2019. Your strength, love, and resilience continue to inspire me every day. This story is for you and for all the families who face the challenges of neurodegenerative diseases with courage and hope. Your legacy lives on in every word, every page, and every heart touched by this book.

CONTENTS

This book, **"A Legacy of Hope: The Journey to Cure PSP and Transform Lives"** is a work of fiction inspired by real-life experiences and the incredible strength of those affected by neurodegenerative diseases. While the characters and events in this story are fictional, they are based on the profound challenges and triumphs faced by countless families around the world.

In crafting this narrative, I have drawn upon the universal themes of love, resilience, and the unyielding human spirit. The Sara Jones Foundation, though a product of imagination, represents the very real efforts of organizations and individuals who dedicate their lives to supporting those in need, advancing medical research, and advocating for better care and understanding of neurological conditions.

This story is a tribute to the courage of those who navigate the difficult journey of Progressive Supranuclear Palsy (PSP) and other neurodegenerative diseases. It is a testament to the power of community, the importance of innovative research, and the enduring impact of a mother's love.

As you read, I hope you find inspiration in the fictional journey of Chrissy and the Sara Jones Foundation. May it remind you of the extraordinary potential within each of us to make a difference, no matter the obstacles we face.

Thank you for joining me on this journey of hope, compassion, and unwavering determination.

Chapter 1: A Subtle Thief

The sun filtered through the lace curtains, casting a warm glow over the living room where Sara Jones sat, her knitting needles clacking rhythmically. She was a picture of serene concentration, her grey hair pulled back into a neat bun. To the casual observer, everything seemed perfectly normal. But to those who knew her well, a shadow was beginning to form.

Sara's daughter, Chrissy, watched from the kitchen, her heart heavy with a mix of love and concern. She noticed the slight tremor in her mother's hands, the way her once nimble fingers occasionally fumbled with the yarn. It was subtle, almost imperceptible, but Chrissy had seen it. It was the first hint of something that would soon become undeniable.

"Mom, do you need anything?" Chrissy called out, trying to keep her voice light and cheerful.

Sara looked up, her eyes twinkling with affection. "No, dear, I'm fine. Just working on this scarf for your father. It's his favourite colour, you know."

Chrissy smiled, though it didn't quite reach her eyes. "Yes, I know. He'll love it."

As the days turned into weeks, the small changes in Sara became more frequent. She began to have difficulty with tasks she had always performed effortlessly. Simple movements required more concentration, and there were moments when her eyes seemed to struggle to track objects or people.

One afternoon, while out for their usual walk in the park, Chrissy noticed her mother's steps becoming hesitant. Sara, who once walked with a brisk, confident stride, now seemed to shuffle, her feet dragging slightly on the pavement. Chrissy gently took her mother's arm, offering support without making it obvious.

"Are you feeling okay, Mom?" she asked, her voice tinged with worry.

Sara sighed, a small frown creasing her forehead. "Just a bit tired, dear. Maybe we should head back."

Chrissy nodded, masking her growing unease. She decided it was time to see a doctor. The appointment was made, and they visited Dr. Thompson, a neurologist with a kind demeanour and a reputation for thoroughness.

Dr. Thompson conducted a series of tests, his expression growing more serious with each passing minute. Finally, he sat them down in his office, the air thick with unspoken fears.

"Mrs. Jones, Chrissy," he began, choosing his words carefully, "I believe you may be experiencing symptoms of Progressive Supranuclear Palsy, or PSP. It's a rare neurological disorder that affects movement, balance, and eye coordination."

Chrissy felt a chill run down her spine. The words sounded foreign, menacing. "What does this mean for my mom?" she asked, her voice barely above a whisper.

Dr. Thompson explained the condition, its symptoms, and the prognosis. PSP was progressive, with no known cure. It would slowly but inexorably steal away Sara's physical abilities, though her mind would remain sharp for much longer.

Sara listened quietly, her face a mask of calm. When Dr. Thompson finished, she reached over and took Chrissy's hand, giving it a reassuring squeeze. "We'll get through this, sweetheart," she said, her voice steady. "We've faced challenges before, and we'll face this one together."

The days that followed were a blur of appointments, physical therapy sessions, and adjustments to their daily routine. Sara's condition progressed, but she faced it with grace and determination. Chrissy became her mother's advocate, learning everything she could about PSP, seeking out the best treatments and support systems.

Together, they navigated the uncertain terrain of this new reality, their bond growing stronger with each passing day. It was a journey marked by small victories and inevitable setbacks, but through it all, they remained steadfast in their resolve to live each day to the fullest.

And so, the subtle thief that was PSP had entered their lives, but Sara and Chrissy faced it head-on, determined to write their own story of resilience and love.

Chapter 2: The New Normal

Mornings in the Jones household had always been bustling, filled with the sounds of coffee brewing, toast popping, and the hum of daily life. But now, the rhythm had changed. Chrissy had moved back into her childhood home to be closer to her mother, and their mornings were quieter, marked by a new routine.

Chrissy woke early, slipping out of bed and padding softly to the kitchen. She brewed a pot of chamomile tea, knowing it was easier on her mother's stomach than the strong coffee Sara used to prefer. She set out a light breakfast, making sure everything was ready before gently waking her mother.

Sara's mornings were slow, a careful dance of movements to avoid the dizziness and stiffness that often greeted her upon waking. Chrissy helped her dress, choosing soft, comfortable clothes that were easy to manage. Despite the challenges, Sara never lost her grace, her movements deliberate and dignified.

"Good morning, Mom," Chrissy said, her voice warm as she entered her mother's room. "I made your favorite toast with a bit of honey."

Sara smiled, her eyes lighting up. "Thank you, dear. It smells wonderful."

They shared breakfast at the kitchen table, talking about the little things that made up their day. Chrissy cherished these moments, finding solace in the simple act of being together.

After breakfast, they prepared for their physical therapy session. Chrissy had found a therapist, Emma, who specialized in neurological conditions. Emma visited the house three times a week, guiding Sara through exercises designed to maintain her strength and balance for as long as possible.

"Good morning, Sara, Chrissy," Emma greeted them with a smile. "Ready for our session today?"

Sara nodded, determination in her eyes. "Always."

They worked through a series of exercises, Chrissy assisting when needed. She watched as her mother focused intently, her determination unwavering even when her body refused to cooperate. Emma was patient and encouraging, praising each small victory.

"You're doing great, Sara," Emma said, helping her back to her chair. "Remember, it's not about how fast you go, but that you keep moving."

Sara nodded, catching her breath. "Thank you, Emma. I won't give up."

As the days turned into weeks, Chrissy and Sara settled into their new normal. Chrissy adjusted her work schedule, balancing her career with caring for her mother. She set up a small office in the corner of the living room, where she could work remotely and still be close by.

Evenings were spent together, watching old movies or reading books. Sara's love for literature remained undiminished, and they often read aloud to each other, sharing favorite passages and discussing the stories. It was a way to escape, to find solace in the worlds created by their favorite authors.

One evening, as they sat together on the couch, Chrissy turned to her mother. "Mom, I've been thinking about starting a foundation.

Something to raise awareness about PSP and support families going through what we are. What do you think?"

Sara's eyes sparkled with pride. "I think it's a wonderful idea, Chrissy. So many people need help and understanding. If our experience can make a difference, then it's worth it."

Chrissy felt a swell of emotion. "I want to name it after you, Mom. The Sara Jones Foundation. To honor your strength and resilience."

Sara reached over, taking her daughter's hand. "Thank you, Chrissy. It means the world to me."

And so, amidst the challenges and adjustments, a new purpose began to take shape. Chrissy threw herself into the creation of the foundation, drawing on her professional skills and personal experiences. She reached out to doctors, therapists, and families, building a network of support and resources.

The Sara Jones Foundation became a beacon of hope for those affected by PSP, offering information, assistance, and a sense of community. Chrissy's dedication and Sara's spirit infused the foundation with a unique warmth and authenticity.

Through it all, Chrissy and Sara continued to face each day together, their bond unbreakable. They found strength in each other, navigating the highs and lows with grace and love. And as they moved forward, they knew they were not alone, but part of a larger journey, united by hope and resilience.

Chapter 3: Spreading the Word

The Sara Jones Foundation was officially launched on a crisp autumn day. Chrissy stood before a small crowd gathered at the local community center, her heart pounding with a mix of excitement and nerves. Sara sat in the front row, her presence a source of strength and inspiration.

"Thank you all for coming today," Chrissy began, her voice steady. "The Sara Jones Foundation is dedicated to raising awareness about Progressive Supranuclear Palsy and providing support to families affected by this challenging condition. My mother, Sara, has faced PSP with incredible courage, and it's her strength that has inspired this foundation."

The room erupted in applause, and Chrissy took a moment to let the support wash over her. She shared their journey, the struggles and the small victories, and the vision for the foundation. It was a deeply personal speech, resonating with many in the audience who had faced similar battles.

After the launch event, Chrissy was approached by several people who wanted to get involved. Among them was Dr. Samantha Gray, a neurologist who had dedicated her career to researching PSP and related disorders.

"Chrissy, your speech was incredibly moving," Dr. Gray said, shaking Chrissy's hand. "I'd love to collaborate with the foundation. There's so much we can do together to advance research and support families."

Chrissy felt a surge of hope. "Thank you, Dr. Gray. Your expertise would be invaluable. Let's set up a meeting to discuss how we can work together."

Over the next few weeks, the foundation began to take shape. Chrissy and Dr. Gray organized informational seminars, support groups, and fundraising events. They reached out to the community, spreading awareness about PSP and the resources available through the foundation.

One afternoon, as Chrissy was finalizing details for an upcoming seminar, she received a call from Emma, Sara's physical therapist. Emma's voice was filled with excitement.

"Chrissy, I've been talking to some colleagues, and we think we can start a specialized exercise program for PSP patients through the foundation. It would focus on maintaining mobility and balance, tailored to their specific needs."

Chrissy's eyes lit up. "That's a fantastic idea, Emma! Let's plan a meeting to discuss the logistics. This could make a huge difference for so many people."

As the foundation's activities expanded, Sara remained at the heart of it all. She attended events, spoke with families, and offered her unique perspective on living with PSP. Her presence was a constant reminder of the foundation's mission and the reason behind their work.

One evening, after a particularly successful fundraiser, Chrissy and Sara sat together on the porch, enjoying the cool breeze and the satisfaction of a job well done.

"Mom, I couldn't have done any of this without you," Chrissy said, her voice filled with gratitude. "Your strength keeps me going."

Sara smiled, her eyes reflecting the love she felt for her daughter. "And I couldn't be prouder of you, Chrissy. You've turned our struggle into something that's helping so many people. That's a true gift."

As the seasons changed, so did the foundation. It grew, encompassing new programs and reaching more families. Chrissy's dedication was unwavering, fueled by the deep bond she shared with her mother and the desire to make a difference.

One day, as Chrissy was preparing for a radio interview to promote the foundation, she received a message from Dr. Gray. It was about a promising new research study on PSP treatments.

"Chrissy, this study could be a game-changer," Dr. Gray wrote. "If the foundation can help fund it, we might be able to accelerate the development of new therapies."

Chrissy felt a rush of excitement. She immediately scheduled a meeting with Dr. Gray to discuss how they could support the study. The possibility of contributing to a breakthrough in PSP research was exactly the kind of impact she had hoped for when starting the foundation.

The radio interview went well, with Chrissy eloquently sharing their story and the foundation's mission. She emphasized the importance of research and the need for community support, urging listeners to get involved.

As she left the studio, her phone buzzed with messages of support and interest. It was clear that the foundation was resonating with people, touching hearts and inspiring action.

Back at home, Chrissy found Sara in the garden, tending to her beloved roses. Despite the challenges of PSP, Sara had never given up her passion for gardening. It was her sanctuary, a place where she felt connected to life's beauty and resilience.

"Mom, the interview went great," Chrissy said, joining her by the roses. "And Dr. Gray has some exciting news about a new research study. The foundation might be able to help fund it."

Sara looked up, her face lighting up with hope. "That's wonderful, Chrissy. Every step forward is a step closer to making a difference."

Chrissy nodded, feeling a renewed sense of purpose. Together, they would continue to fight, to spread awareness, and to support others on this journey. The foundation was more than just an organization; it was a testament to their love and determination.

And so, they moved forward, hand in hand, their hearts full of hope and their eyes set on a brighter future. The subtle thief that was PSP might have changed their lives, but it could never diminish their spirit or their resolve to make the world a better place for those who followed.

Chapter 4: New Horizons

The Sara Jones Foundation had become a well-known entity in the world of neurological disorders, particularly in the realm of PSP. With their growing influence, Chrissy and her team began to explore new horizons. They reached out to international researchers and organizations, forging partnerships that would further their mission.

One of the foundation's biggest breakthroughs came when Dr. Gray secured a partnership with a renowned research institute in Europe. The institute was on the cutting edge of neurological research, and their collaboration opened up new possibilities for finding a cure for PSP.

"Chrissy, this partnership could accelerate our research by years," Dr. Gray said during one of their meetings. "They have access to technology and resources that we can only dream of."

Chrissy felt a surge of hope. "This is exactly what we need, Dr. Gray. Let's make sure we give them all the support they need from our end."

With the new partnership in place, the foundation launched an ambitious fundraising campaign to support the joint research project. Chrissy traveled across the country, speaking at conferences and events, sharing their story, and rallying support.

During one of these trips, she met David, a tech entrepreneur who had lost his father to PSP. David was deeply moved by Chrissy's dedication and offered to help the foundation with his expertise in technology and innovation.

"Chrissy, I believe in what you're doing," David said. "I want to help you take this foundation to the next level. Let's leverage technology to reach more people and raise more awareness."

Chrissy was thrilled by the offer. With David's help, they revamped the foundation's website, created an app for patients and caregivers, and used social media to spread their message more effectively. The impact was immediate and profound. More people than ever before were engaging with the foundation, seeking help, and offering support.

Back home, Sara watched the progress with pride and joy. Despite her condition, she remained an active part of the foundation, offering her insights and encouragement.

One evening, as they were preparing for bed, Sara turned to Chrissy. "You've done so much, Chrissy. You've given me and so many others hope."

Chrissy hugged her mother tightly. "We've done this together, Mom. Your strength inspires me every day."

The foundation's efforts began to pay off. The research collaboration yielded promising results, and new therapies were being developed. Patients and families found solace and support through the foundation's programs, and the awareness about PSP grew exponentially.

One day, as Chrissy was reviewing the latest research reports, she received a call from Dr. Gray. Her voice was filled with excitement.

"Chrissy, we've made a breakthrough," Dr. Gray said. "The new therapy is showing remarkable results in our trials. It's not a cure, but it's a significant step forward."

Tears filled Chrissy's eyes. "That's incredible, Dr. Gray. This is what we've been working towards. Thank you for everything."

As she hung up the phone, Chrissy felt a profound sense of accomplishment. The journey had been long and challenging, but they were making a difference. She went to find Sara, who was sitting in the garden, enjoying the afternoon sun.

"Mom, we've got good news," Chrissy said, her voice trembling with emotion. "The new therapy is working. We're making progress."

Sara's eyes filled with tears of joy. "I knew we could do it, Chrissy. I never doubted it for a moment."

And so, they continued their journey, fueled by hope and determination. The Sara Jones Foundation had become a beacon of light for those affected by PSP, and their work was far from over. Together, Chrissy and Sara, along with their dedicated team, would keep pushing forward, making the world a better place, one step at a time.

Chapter 5: The Impact Grows

The Sara Jones Foundation's success continued to build momentum, and with it came an influx of opportunities and challenges. Chrissy found herself busier than ever, balancing her time between managing the foundation's day-to-day operations and strategizing for its future growth.

One sunny afternoon, Chrissy received a call from a major pharmaceutical company interested in collaborating on the development of new treatments for PSP. The company's interest represented a significant milestone for the foundation, marking its influence in the broader medical community.

"We've been following your work, Chrissy," said Dr. Martin, the company's lead researcher, during their first meeting. "Your foundation has created an incredible network of support and awareness. We believe that, together, we can accelerate the development of effective treatments for PSP."

Chrissy felt a surge of excitement. "Thank you, Dr. Martin. This partnership could be transformative for our work. We're committed to finding better treatments and, ultimately, a cure for PSP."

The partnership brought new resources and expertise to the foundation, allowing them to expand their research and support initiatives. Chrissy worked closely with Dr. Martin and his team, ensuring that the foundation's goals and values were at the forefront of their collaboration.

Back at home, Sara's condition had stabilized thanks to the new therapy. While she still faced daily challenges, the progress was undeniable. She continued to be an active participant in the foundation's activities, her spirit and resilience serving as a source of inspiration for everyone involved.

One evening, as Chrissy and Sara sat on the porch watching the sunset, Sara turned to her daughter with a thoughtful expression.

"Chrissy, I've been thinking about our journey," Sara said. "We've come so far, and I'm so proud of everything you've accomplished. But I want to make sure that the foundation continues to thrive, even after I'm gone."

Chrissy's eyes filled with tears. "Mom, don't talk like that. You're still here with us, and you're still fighting."

Sara squeezed her daughter's hand. "I know, sweetheart. But we have to plan for the future. I want to establish an endowment fund for the foundation, something that will ensure its work continues for generations to come."

Chrissy nodded, understanding the wisdom in her mother's words. "You're right, Mom. We'll start working on it right away."

With renewed determination, Chrissy and the foundation's board set to work on creating the Sara Jones Endowment Fund. They reached out to donors, held fundraising events, and spread the word about their long-term vision. The response was overwhelming, with supporters eager to contribute to the foundation's lasting legacy.

As the endowment fund grew, so did the foundation's impact. They were able to launch new programs, including a scholarship fund for medical students pursuing research in neurological disorders and a grant program for families affected by PSP to cover medical and living expenses.

One day, Chrissy received an email from a young researcher named Dr. Aisha Malik, who had recently completed her PhD in neuroscience. Dr. Malik was passionate about PSP research and had developed a promising new approach to understanding the disease's progression.

"Chrissy, I've been following the Sara Jones Foundation for years, and your work has been a huge inspiration for me," Dr. Malik wrote. "I would love to join your team and contribute to your research efforts."

Chrissy was thrilled. Dr. Malik's expertise and fresh perspective were exactly what the foundation needed. She quickly arranged a meeting, and it wasn't long before Dr. Malik became a key member of their research team.

With Dr. Malik on board, the foundation's research efforts took a significant leap forward. They began exploring innovative therapies and potential treatments, driven by a shared commitment to making a difference.

As the foundation continued to grow, so did its influence. The Sara Jones Foundation became a leading voice in the fight against PSP, advocating for better healthcare policies and increased funding for neurological research. They organized conferences and symposiums, bringing together experts from around the world to share knowledge and collaborate.

One such conference was held in New York City, drawing attendees from across the globe. Chrissy stood before a packed auditorium, feeling a mix of pride and humility as she addressed the crowd.

"Thank you all for being here today," she began. "When we started the Sara Jones Foundation, our goal was to make a difference in the lives of those affected by PSP. Today, we're not just making a difference; we're driving change, fostering innovation, and building a community of hope and support."

The audience erupted in applause, and Chrissy felt a deep sense of fulfillment. The foundation had come a long way from its humble beginnings, but their mission remained the same: to honor Sara's legacy and to fight for a future free from PSP.

As the conference concluded, Chrissy and her team received numerous offers of collaboration and support from organizations and researchers eager to join their cause. The foundation's network continued to expand, and their impact reached further than ever before.

Back home, Sara watched the news coverage of the conference with tears of joy in her eyes. Despite the challenges she faced, she knew that their work was making a real difference in the world. She felt a deep sense of peace, knowing that the foundation would continue to thrive and grow, driven by the love and determination of her daughter and the countless others who believed in their mission.

And so, the Sara Jones Foundation continued to forge ahead, fueled by hope, resilience, and an unwavering commitment to a brighter future. Together, they faced each new challenge with courage and compassion, knowing that every step forward brought them closer to a world where PSP was no longer a devastating diagnosis, but a condition that could be understood, treated, and ultimately, cured.

Chapter 6: A Beacon of Hope

The Sara Jones Foundation had grown into a beacon of hope and a model for other organizations focused on rare neurological diseases. With their successful partnerships and the establishment of the Sara Jones Endowment Fund, the foundation was well-equipped to make long-term impacts.

One morning, Chrissy received a call from a well-known philanthropist, Grace Williams. Grace had been moved by the foundation's story and wanted to discuss a potential multi-million-dollar donation.

"Chrissy, I've followed your work for some time now," Grace said warmly. "The way you've built this foundation in honor of your mother is truly inspiring. I want to help you take it even further."

Chrissy felt a surge of gratitude. "Thank you so much, Grace. Your support could open so many new doors for us. We have big plans for the future, and with your help, we can achieve them."

The donation from Grace Williams allowed the foundation to launch several new initiatives, including a global awareness campaign and a state-of-the-art research lab dedicated to PSP and related disorders. The lab attracted top scientists from around the world, all eager to contribute to the groundbreaking work being done.

In the midst of these advancements, Chrissy received an unexpected message from an old friend, Mark, who had lost touch over the years. He had seen a news segment about the foundation and reached out to reconnect.

"Chrissy, it's been too long," Mark wrote. "I'm so proud of everything you've accomplished. I'd love to catch up and see how I can support your efforts."

Chrissy was delighted to hear from Mark. They met for coffee and reminisced about old times, sharing updates on their lives. Mark, now a successful lawyer, offered his services to the foundation pro bono, helping them navigate the legal aspects of their expansion.

With Mark's legal expertise, the foundation established several international branches, extending their reach and impact globally. They launched educational programs in developing countries, ensuring that families and healthcare providers had access to vital information about PSP.

During one of her trips to establish a new branch in India, Chrissy met Dr. Rajiv Patel, a neurologist with a deep commitment to improving the lives of those affected by neurological disorders. Dr. Patel's innovative approach to patient care and community outreach impressed Chrissy, and she invited him to join the foundation's advisory board.

"Your work here is incredible, Dr. Patel," Chrissy said during their meeting. "We would be honored to have you on our team and help guide our efforts globally."

Dr. Patel accepted the invitation with enthusiasm, bringing his wealth of experience and passion to the foundation. Under his guidance, they developed culturally sensitive programs that addressed the unique challenges faced by patients and families in different parts of the world.

Back in the United States, Sara continued to be a pillar of strength and inspiration. Her resilience and positive outlook touched everyone she met, and her story was frequently shared at foundation events and conferences.

One day, as Chrissy and Sara sat in the garden, Sara turned to her daughter with a contented smile.

"Chrissy, I'm so proud of you," Sara said softly. "You've built something truly remarkable. I feel at peace knowing that our work will continue to help so many people."

Chrissy hugged her mother tightly. "Thank you, Mom. None of this would have been possible without your strength and courage. You're the heart of this foundation."

As the foundation continued to grow, Chrissy received an invitation to speak at a prestigious international medical conference in Geneva. The conference brought together leading experts in neurology, and Chrissy's keynote address was a highlight of the event.

"Good afternoon, everyone," Chrissy began, standing before an audience of esteemed colleagues. "The Sara Jones Foundation started as a tribute to my mother's strength and resilience. Today, it's a global movement dedicated to fighting PSP and improving the lives of those affected by neurological disorders. Our journey has been one of hope, collaboration, and unwavering determination."

The audience listened intently as Chrissy shared the foundation's accomplishments and future goals. Her speech was met with a standing ovation, and many attendees expressed interest in collaborating with the foundation.

Following the conference, Chrissy met with Dr. Elena Rossi, a leading researcher in neurodegenerative diseases. Dr. Rossi had developed a cutting-edge gene therapy technique that showed promise for treating PSP.

"Chrissy, your foundation's work is extraordinary," Dr. Rossi said. "I believe my research could greatly benefit from your support and resources. Together, we could make significant strides in treating PSP."

Chrissy was excited about the potential collaboration. "Dr. Rossi, your work is exactly the kind of innovative approach we're looking for. Let's discuss how we can support each other and move forward with this promising research."

Back at the foundation's headquarters, the team was buzzing with excitement about the new developments. The research lab was bustling with activity, and the global awareness campaign was reaching millions of people. The foundation's website and app provided a wealth of resources, and their support programs were making a tangible difference in the lives of patients and families.

As the years passed, the Sara Jones Foundation continued to be a beacon of hope and progress. Chrissy and her team remained dedicated to their mission, driven by the love and resilience that had started it all. They knew that every step forward brought them closer to a future where PSP was no longer a devastating diagnosis but a condition that could be understood, treated, and ultimately, cured.

Through it all, Sara's spirit remained a guiding light, reminding them of the power of love, determination, and the unbreakable bond between a mother and her daughter. Together, they faced each new challenge with courage and compassion, knowing that their work was making a profound difference in the world.

Chapter 7: A Legacy of Love

The seasons changed, and with them came the inevitable progression of Sara's condition. Despite the new therapies and treatments, PSP continued its relentless course. Sara's strength and resilience were unwavering, but Chrissy could see the toll it was taking on her mother.

One crisp autumn morning, Chrissy noticed that Sara seemed unusually tired. She moved slower, and her usually bright eyes were clouded with fatigue.

"Mom, how are you feeling today?" Chrissy asked gently as she helped her mother to her favorite chair by the window.

Sara gave her a weak smile. "Just a bit more tired than usual, sweetheart. I think I'll rest here for a while."

Chrissy nodded, her heart heavy with unspoken worry. She spent the day close by, attending to her mother's needs and savoring every moment they had together.

As the days turned into weeks, Sara's condition continued to decline. The once vibrant woman who had been the heart and soul of the Sara Jones Foundation was now facing her final days with grace and dignity. Chrissy stayed by her side, providing comfort and care, cherishing their remaining time together.

One quiet evening, as the first snowflakes of winter began to fall, Sara called Chrissy to her bedside.

"Chrissy," Sara said softly, her voice barely above a whisper. "I want you to promise me something."

Chrissy held her mother's hand, tears welling in her eyes. "Anything, Mom."

"Promise me that you'll continue our work," Sara said, her eyes filled with love and determination. "Promise me that you'll keep fighting for a cure, for better treatments, and for all the families affected by PSP."

Chrissy nodded, her voice choked with emotion. "I promise, Mom. I'll continue our work and make sure your legacy lives on."

Sara smiled, a peaceful look settling over her face. "I know you will, Chrissy. You've made me so proud."

That night, Sara passed away quietly in her sleep, surrounded by love and the profound impact she had made on the world.

The days that followed were filled with a deep sense of loss and mourning. The foundation's staff, volunteers, and supporters rallied around Chrissy, offering their condolences and sharing stories of how Sara had touched their lives.

A memorial service was held to celebrate Sara's life and legacy. People from all walks of life attended, each with their own story of how Sara had inspired them. Chrissy stood before the gathering, her heart heavy but her resolve stronger than ever.

"Today, we honor the life of an incredible woman," Chrissy began, her voice steady. "Sara Jones was more than just my mother; she was a beacon of hope and resilience for everyone who knew her. Her strength and determination in the face of adversity inspired us all, and her legacy will continue to guide our work at the foundation."

As she spoke, Chrissy felt a wave of love and support from the crowd. She knew that her mother's spirit would always be with her, driving her forward in their shared mission.

In the months that followed, the Sara Jones Foundation redoubled its efforts, inspired by Sara's memory. Chrissy and her team launched new initiatives, including a research fellowship in Sara's name, dedicated to advancing the understanding and treatment of PSP. They expanded their support programs, reaching more families than ever before.

One day, Chrissy received a letter from a woman named Maria, whose husband had been diagnosed with PSP. Maria wrote about how the foundation's resources and support had been a lifeline for her family during their darkest times.

"Your mother's story and the work of the foundation have given us hope when we thought there was none," Maria wrote. "Thank you for continuing her legacy and for making a difference in the lives of so many."

Chrissy read the letter with tears in her eyes, her heart filled with gratitude and purpose. She knew that the promise she had made to her mother was not just a commitment to continue their work, but a vow to honor Sara's life by bringing hope and support to those who needed it most.

As the foundation moved forward, Chrissy felt her mother's presence in every step they took. Sara's legacy lived on in the research they funded, the families they helped, and the awareness they raised. Together, they continued to fight for a world where PSP was no longer a devastating diagnosis but a condition that could be understood, treated, and ultimately, cured.

Through the pain of loss and the challenges ahead, Chrissy and the Sara Jones Foundation remained steadfast in their mission. They faced each day with the same strength and resilience that Sara had shown, knowing that her spirit would guide them on their journey.

And so, the story of Sara Jones and her foundation continued, a testament to the power of love, determination, and the enduring impact of one woman's incredible life.

Chapter 8: Continuing the Mission

The Sara Jones Foundation entered a new era, driven by the memory of its namesake and the promise Chrissy had made. The work was more critical than ever, and the foundation's reach continued to grow.

One brisk spring morning, Chrissy sat in her office, surrounded by the vibrant energy of the foundation's bustling headquarters. She was preparing for a significant meeting with government officials to advocate for increased funding for neurological research. The stakes were high, but Chrissy was determined to honor her mother's legacy by securing more resources for the fight against PSP.

As she reviewed her talking points, her phone buzzed with a message from David, the tech entrepreneur who had become a crucial partner and close friend. David had been instrumental in modernizing the foundation's digital presence, helping to amplify their message and connect with a broader audience.

"Good luck today, Chrissy. You've got this. Let's make sure everyone hears Sara's story," the message read.

Chrissy smiled, drawing strength from David's support. She took a deep breath and headed to the meeting, ready to make her case.

The meeting was intense, but Chrissy's passion and dedication shone through. She shared Sara's story, highlighting the impact of the foundation's work and the urgent need for more funding and research.

"We have made significant strides, but there is still so much more to do," Chrissy concluded. "By investing in research and support, we can bring hope to countless families affected by PSP and other neurological disorders. Together, we can honor the legacy of those like my mother, Sara Jones, and create a future where no one has to face this journey alone."

The officials were moved by Chrissy's words, and after a series of follow-up meetings, they announced a substantial increase in funding for neurological research. It was a significant victory, and Chrissy knew it was just the beginning.

Back at the foundation, the news was met with celebration. Chrissy gathered her team for a moment of reflection and gratitude.

"This is a huge step forward," Chrissy said, her voice filled with emotion. "I want to thank each and every one of you for your dedication and hard work. This victory belongs to all of us, and it's a testament to the power of our mission and the legacy of my mother, Sara."

The team applauded, their spirits lifted by the success. But Chrissy knew there was still much work to be done.

As the foundation expanded its efforts, they launched new initiatives to support caregivers and families affected by PSP. One such program was the "Sara's Circle" support groups, which provided a safe space for families to share their experiences, offer each other support, and learn from experts.

During one of these support group meetings, Chrissy met Linda, a young mother whose husband had recently been diagnosed with PSP. Linda was struggling to balance caring for her husband, raising their children, and managing her own career.

"Chrissy, I don't know how you did it," Linda said, tears in her eyes. "Some days, it feels like too much to handle."

Chrissy reached out and took Linda's hand. "I understand, Linda. It's incredibly challenging, but you're not alone. We're here to support you every step of the way. My mother's strength gave me the courage to keep going, and I see that same strength in you."

Linda nodded, finding comfort in Chrissy's words. The support group became a lifeline for her, offering practical advice, emotional support, and a sense of community.

Meanwhile, the foundation's research efforts continued to make strides. Dr. Aisha Malik's innovative work on gene therapy showed promising results, and the team was optimistic about the potential for new treatments. Chrissy regularly visited the research lab, staying updated on their progress and offering her encouragement.

One afternoon, as Chrissy walked through the lab, Dr. Malik approached her with a look of excitement.

"Chrissy, we've just completed a successful trial with our latest gene therapy technique," Dr. Malik said. "The results are incredibly promising. We're seeing significant improvements in patients' motor functions and quality of life."

Chrissy felt a surge of hope. "That's amazing news, Dr. Malik. Your work is changing lives, and I know my mother would be so proud of what we're accomplishing."

The breakthrough was a turning point for the foundation. They began preparing for larger clinical trials, working closely with regulatory agencies and medical institutions. The promise of a new, effective treatment for PSP was within reach, and the foundation's efforts were gaining international recognition.

As the foundation celebrated these milestones, Chrissy took a moment to reflect on their journey. She visited her mother's favorite spot in the garden, sitting quietly among the blooming roses that Sara had lovingly tended.

"Mom, we're making progress," Chrissy whispered, feeling a deep connection to her mother. "Your strength and spirit are with us every step of the way. We're going to make a difference, just like you wanted."

The foundation's impact continued to grow, reaching more people and making tangible improvements in the lives of those affected by PSP. Chrissy knew that the road ahead would still have its challenges, but she was ready to face them with the same determination and resilience that had guided her from the beginning.

And so, the Sara Jones Foundation moved forward, a testament to the power of love, hope, and the enduring legacy of an extraordinary woman. Through their work, they honored Sara's memory and brought hope to countless families, driven by a mission that would continue to inspire and transform lives for generations to come.

Chapter 9: Creating Moments of Joy

The Sara Jones Foundation had always focused on providing support and hope to families affected by PSP. As they continued to expand their efforts, Chrissy and her team brainstormed new ways to bring relief and joy to those navigating this challenging journey.

One afternoon, during a meeting with the foundation's board of directors, Chrissy shared an idea that had been on her mind for some time.

"I've been thinking about how we can offer more than just medical and emotional support," Chrissy began. "What if we could provide families with an opportunity to take a break from their daily struggles and create lasting memories together? I'm envisioning a program that offers respite vacations for families affected by PSP."

The room buzzed with excitement as the board members discussed the idea. They could see the potential impact of such a program, giving families a chance to relax and enjoy quality time without the constant stress of caregiving.

"That's a wonderful idea, Chrissy," said David, the tech entrepreneur. "We could partner with resorts and travel companies to make this happen. It would be a beautiful way to honor Sara's legacy and bring joy to these families."

With unanimous support from the board, Chrissy and her team set to work on developing the program, which they named "Sara's

Retreats." The goal was to provide all-expenses-paid vacations to serene destinations where families could recharge and create cherished memories together.

They reached out to potential partners, including travel agencies, hotels, and resorts. Many were eager to join the cause, inspired by the foundation's mission and the heartfelt story behind it. Within a few months, the first Sara's Retreats were ready to launch.

To select the families, the foundation opened an application process, encouraging caregivers to share their stories and explain how a respite vacation would benefit their loved ones. The response was overwhelming, with many heartfelt and moving applications pouring in.

One of the first families chosen for the program was the Martinez family. Maria Martinez had written a touching letter about her husband, Carlos, who had been diagnosed with PSP two years earlier. The family had been struggling to balance Carlos's care with raising their two young children, and a vacation seemed like an impossible dream.

When Chrissy called Maria to share the news, the response was emotional.

"Maria, I'm thrilled to let you know that your family has been selected for Sara's Retreats," Chrissy said warmly. "We're sending you to a beautiful resort where you can relax and make wonderful memories together."

Maria's voice trembled with gratitude. "Thank you so much, Chrissy. This means the world to us. Carlos and the kids will be overjoyed. We really needed this."

The foundation covered all expenses, including travel, accommodation, and special activities tailored to the family's needs. For the Martinez family, the destination was a tranquil beach resort, complete with accessible amenities and a variety of activities to ensure everyone could enjoy their time.

As the family arrived at the resort, they were greeted with warm smiles and personalized welcome packages. The children's faces lit up with excitement as they explored the beautiful surroundings, while Carlos and Maria felt a wave of relief wash over them.

During their stay, the Martinez family enjoyed a range of activities, from beach outings to family-friendly excursions. There were moments of laughter and joy, simple pleasures that had been overshadowed by the daily challenges of PSP. Maria and Carlos cherished quiet evenings together, watching the sunset and feeling a renewed sense of connection and hope.

Back at the foundation, Chrissy received photos and messages from the Martinez family, sharing their experiences and expressing their heartfelt thanks.

"Chrissy, this trip has been a gift beyond words," Maria wrote. "We've created so many wonderful memories, and it's given us the strength to keep going. Thank you for making this possible."

The success of the first Sara's Retreats inspired Chrissy and her team to expand the program further. They continued to partner with more resorts and travel companies, ensuring that more families could benefit from these respite vacations. The stories of joy and renewal from the participating families fueled their commitment to growing the initiative.

One evening, as Chrissy reviewed the latest batch of applications, she felt a deep sense of fulfillment. Sara's Retreats had become a powerful way to honor her mother's legacy, bringing moments of joy and relief to families who needed it most.

Chrissy decided to visit one of the retreats herself, joining a group of families at a mountain resort. As she spent time with them, she witnessed firsthand the transformative impact of the program. She saw families laughing together, sharing meals, and simply enjoying each other's company without the constant burden of caregiving.

During a campfire gathering, one of the parents, John, approached Chrissy with tears in his eyes.

"Chrissy, I can't thank you enough for this," John said, his voice filled with emotion. "This retreat has given us a sense of normalcy that we haven't felt in a long time. It's reminded us of the joy and love that PSP can't take away."

Chrissy hugged John, feeling a deep connection to the families she had met. "I'm so glad to hear that, John. This is exactly why we started Sara's Retreats. We want to give you these precious moments, because every family deserves to make beautiful memories together."

As the retreat came to an end, Chrissy reflected on the journey that had brought them here. The Sara Jones Foundation had grown into a force for good, touching lives in ways she had never imagined. And through it all, the spirit of her mother, Sara, remained a guiding light, inspiring every step they took.

With Sara's Retreats, the foundation had found a new way to bring hope and happiness to families affected by PSP. Chrissy knew that as they continued to expand the program, they would create even more moments of joy, helping families build memories that would last a lifetime.

And so, the Sara Jones Foundation continued its mission, driven by love, resilience, and the enduring legacy of an extraordinary woman. Through their work, they brought light to the darkest days, offering hope, support, and the chance to create moments of pure, unfiltered joy.

Chapter 10: A Sanctuary in the Caribbean

The success of Sara's Retreats inspired Chrissy and her team to think even bigger. They had seen firsthand the profound impact that respite vacations had on families affected by PSP, and they wanted to create a more permanent sanctuary where these families could find comprehensive care and relaxation.

One sunny afternoon, during a brainstorming session at the foundation's headquarters, Chrissy proposed an ambitious new idea.

"What if we could open a respite hospice in the Caribbean?" Chrissy suggested. "A place where families can receive both medical care and enjoy a peaceful, beautiful environment. It would be a sanctuary for those who need a break from their daily challenges."

The idea was met with enthusiasm from the board members. The Caribbean offered the perfect setting, with its serene beaches and warm climate, to create a place of healing and tranquility.

David, the tech entrepreneur, immediately saw the potential. "Chrissy, this could be groundbreaking. We could partner with local healthcare providers and resorts to offer top-notch medical care and a luxurious, relaxing experience."

With the board's approval, Chrissy and her team set to work on making the dream a reality. They began by scouting potential locations, eventually settling on a picturesque island with stunning ocean views and a welcoming community.

Next, they partnered with local healthcare providers, ensuring that the hospice would offer comprehensive medical care, including specialized treatments for PSP. They also collaborated with resort developers to create comfortable, accessible accommodations for families.

The project gained momentum quickly, and within a year, the Sara Jones Respite Hospice was ready to open its doors. The hospice was a beautiful blend of medical facility and luxury resort, designed to provide both care and comfort.

The opening ceremony was a grand event, attended by supporters, healthcare professionals, and families affected by PSP. Chrissy stood before the gathering, her heart filled with pride and gratitude.

"Welcome, everyone, to the Sara Jones Respite Hospice," Chrissy began, her voice resonating with emotion. "This sanctuary is a testament to the enduring spirit of my mother, Sara, and to all the families who have inspired us with their strength and resilience. Here, you will find not just medical care, but a place to rest, relax, and create beautiful memories together."

The audience erupted in applause, and Chrissy felt a deep sense of fulfillment. She knew that this hospice would change lives, offering a unique blend of medical support and emotional rejuvenation.

Among the first families to stay at the hospice was the Harris family. John Harris, diagnosed with PSP three years ago, had been struggling with the progression of the disease. His wife, Emily, and their two children were exhausted from the relentless caregiving and the emotional toll it took on them.

When Chrissy greeted the Harris family at the hospice, she saw the relief and hope in their eyes.

"Welcome to our sanctuary," Chrissy said warmly. "We're here to take care of you, so you can focus on spending quality time together."

During their stay, the Harris family enjoyed the hospice's many amenities, from relaxing beachside cabanas to guided meditation sessions. John received expert medical care, while Emily and the children participated in therapeutic activities designed to reduce stress and promote well-being.

One evening, as they watched the sunset from a tranquil garden, John turned to Chrissy with tears in his eyes.

"Chrissy, this place is a gift," John said, his voice filled with gratitude. "For the first time in a long time, we've been able to just be a family, without the constant worry and exhaustion. Thank you for making this possible."

Chrissy felt a lump in her throat. "It's our honor, John. Seeing your family find peace and joy here is exactly why we created this hospice. Your strength and love inspire us every day."

As word of the hospice spread, more families from around the world came to experience its healing environment. The combination of medical care and the serene Caribbean setting provided a unique respite for those facing the challenges of PSP.

Back at the foundation's headquarters, Chrissy and her team continued to innovate, seeking new ways to support their mission. They launched a fundraising campaign to expand the hospice, adding more accommodations and specialized treatment facilities. The response was overwhelming, with donors eager to contribute to such a meaningful cause.

One day, as Chrissy reviewed plans for the expansion, she received a call from Dr. Elena Rossi, the leading researcher in neurodegenerative diseases who had collaborated with the foundation.

"Chrissy, I have exciting news," Dr. Rossi said. "We've developed a new therapy that shows significant promise for slowing the progression of PSP. I'd love to conduct a clinical trial at your hospice, where patients can receive this cutting-edge treatment in a supportive environment."

Chrissy's heart raced with excitement. "That's incredible, Dr. Rossi. Let's make it happen. Our hospice is the perfect place to offer this therapy, combining medical care with a peaceful, healing atmosphere."

The clinical trial brought new hope to families, offering them access to the latest advancements in PSP treatment. The hospice became a hub of innovation and compassion, where science and humanity came together to make a difference.

One evening, as Chrissy walked along the beach, she reflected on the journey that had brought them here. The Sara Jones Foundation had grown beyond her wildest dreams, driven by a mission of love and resilience. The respite hospice in the Caribbean was a shining example of what could be achieved when people came together with a shared purpose.

Chrissy knew that her mother's spirit was with her, guiding every step. She felt a profound sense of peace, knowing that they were making a lasting impact on the lives of families affected by PSP.

As the sun dipped below the horizon, Chrissy made a silent promise to continue their work, to keep pushing forward, and to bring hope to those who needed it most. The Sara Jones Respite Hospice was just the beginning of a new chapter, one filled with compassion, innovation, and the enduring legacy of an extraordinary woman.

Chapter 11: Expanding Horizons

The Sara Jones Respite Hospice in the Caribbean had quickly become a beacon of hope and renewal for families affected by PSP. Its success inspired Chrissy and her team to think about further expanding their reach and impact. They began to explore new horizons, considering how they could bring similar sanctuaries to other parts of the world.

One sunny afternoon, Chrissy sat in her office, brainstorming with David, Dr. Elena Rossi, and a few key members of the foundation's board.

"We've seen how transformative the hospice in the Caribbean has been," Chrissy began. "But there are families all over the world who need this kind of support. I think it's time we consider opening more respite hospices in other regions."

David nodded enthusiastically. "I agree. We've received numerous inquiries from families in Europe, Asia, and Africa, asking if we have similar facilities closer to them. We need to meet this global demand."

Dr. Rossi added, "And from a research perspective, expanding our hospices would allow us to conduct more widespread clinical trials, gathering diverse data that could accelerate the development of new therapies."

With a shared vision, the team set out to identify potential locations for new hospices. They considered areas where access to comprehensive PSP care was limited and where families could benefit most from the foundation's unique blend of medical support and restful environments.

After months of research and planning, they decided to establish new hospices in three key regions: Europe, Southeast Asia, and South America. Each location was chosen for its natural beauty, accessibility, and the potential to build partnerships with local healthcare providers.

The first new hospice was planned for the picturesque countryside of Tuscany, Italy. The serene landscapes, combined with Italy's strong healthcare infrastructure, made it an ideal location. Chrissy traveled to Tuscany to oversee the project, working closely with local officials and medical professionals to ensure the hospice met the highest standards of care and comfort.

During the grand opening of the Tuscan hospice, Chrissy addressed a crowd of supporters, families, and dignitaries.

"Welcome to the Sara Jones Respite Hospice of Tuscany," Chrissy began, her voice filled with emotion. "This sanctuary is a testament to our commitment to bringing hope and healing to families affected by PSP. We are honored to be part of this beautiful community and to extend our mission across the globe."

The Tuscan hospice quickly became a haven for families from across Europe. They enjoyed the peaceful surroundings, gourmet Italian cuisine, and personalized care. The feedback was overwhelmingly positive, with many families expressing gratitude for the respite and rejuvenation the hospice provided.

Next, the foundation turned its attention to Southeast Asia, choosing the tropical island of Bali, Indonesia, for their second new hospice. Bali's natural beauty and rich cultural heritage offered a perfect setting for healing and relaxation. The foundation partnered with local resorts and healthcare providers, creating a sanctuary that blended traditional Balinese wellness practices with modern medical care.

Chrissy visited Bali for the hospice's opening ceremony, feeling a deep sense of connection to the island's tranquil atmosphere.

"Bali is a place of healing and spiritual renewal," Chrissy said during her speech. "Our hope is that the Sara Jones Respite Hospice here will offer families the peace and support they need to navigate their journey with PSP."

The Balinese hospice quickly gained a reputation for its holistic approach to care, incorporating yoga, meditation, and traditional healing practices into the treatment plans. Families from across Asia found solace in the hospice's serene environment, building cherished memories together.

The final location for the new hospices was in the vibrant city of Rio de Janeiro, Brazil. The foundation chose Rio for its stunning beaches, welcoming culture, and the need for specialized PSP care in South America. The Rio hospice featured a blend of medical excellence and the lively spirit of the Brazilian community.

At the opening ceremony in Rio, Chrissy was joined by local officials, healthcare providers, and families eager to experience the new hospice.

"We are thrilled to bring the Sara Jones Respite Hospice to South America," Chrissy said, addressing the crowd. "This hospice embodies our mission to provide care, comfort, and joy to families facing the challenges of PSP. We are honored to be part of this vibrant community."

The Rio hospice quickly became a beloved addition to the foundation's network, offering families a unique blend of medical care and cultural experiences. The hospices in Tuscany, Bali, and Rio all operated with the same core values: compassion, excellence, and the creation of lasting memories.

Back at the foundation's headquarters, Chrissy and her team reflected on the incredible journey they had undertaken. The expansion of the respite hospices was a monumental achievement, made possible by the dedication and support of their global community.

One evening, as Chrissy sat on the porch of the original Caribbean hospice, she felt a deep sense of fulfillment. The foundation had grown beyond her wildest dreams, driven by the love and resilience of countless families and supporters.

Chrissy knew that their work was far from over. There were still many families who needed their help, many lives to touch, and many memories to create. But she felt confident that with the foundation's unwavering commitment and the enduring spirit of her mother, Sara, they could continue to make a difference.

As the sun set over the tranquil waters, Chrissy made a silent vow to keep pushing forward, to keep expanding their horizons, and to keep bringing hope and healing to families around the world. The Sara Jones Foundation had become a global force for good, and its mission to honor Sara's legacy and support families affected by PSP would continue to inspire and transform lives for generations to come.

Chapter 12: A Global Network of Care

With the successful establishment of new respite hospices in Tuscany, Bali, and Rio de Janeiro, the Sara Jones Foundation had truly become a global network of care and support for families affected by PSP. The hospices were thriving, each providing a unique blend of local culture and comprehensive medical care, and the foundation's reach was expanding further than ever before.

One morning, Chrissy received an email from a family in Kenya, sharing their struggles and expressing their desire for similar support in Africa. Touched by their story, Chrissy knew that the foundation's mission needed to extend to this continent as well.

During a board meeting, Chrissy shared the email and proposed the idea of establishing a hospice in Africa.

"Families in Africa face unique challenges when dealing with PSP," Chrissy explained. "We have the opportunity to provide them with the support and resources they desperately need. I believe we should open a respite hospice in Kenya."

The board members agreed, recognizing the importance of expanding their reach to more underserved regions. They began planning for the new hospice, collaborating with local healthcare providers, government officials, and community leaders in Kenya to ensure that the facility would meet the needs of the families it would serve.

After months of preparation, Chrissy and a team from the foundation traveled to Kenya to oversee the project's progress. They selected a beautiful location near Nairobi, surrounded by stunning landscapes and vibrant wildlife. The hospice would offer a peaceful retreat for families while providing top-notch medical care and support.

During the opening ceremony, Chrissy stood before a gathering of families, healthcare professionals, and community members.

"Today, we are honored to open the Sara Jones Respite Hospice in Kenya," Chrissy began, her voice filled with emotion. "This sanctuary is a symbol of our commitment to providing care and support to families affected by PSP, no matter where they are in the world. We are grateful to be part of this wonderful community and look forward to making a positive impact together."

The Kenyan hospice quickly became a haven for families from across Africa. They found solace in the hospice's serene environment and compassionate care, which included access to the latest PSP treatments and therapies. The facility also offered cultural activities, allowing families to connect with Kenya's rich heritage and traditions.

One of the first families to stay at the Kenyan hospice was the Njeri family. Jane Njeri, whose husband, Peter, had been diagnosed with PSP, was overwhelmed with gratitude for the respite the hospice provided.

"Chrissy, this place is a blessing," Jane said, tears of joy in her eyes. "Peter and I have found peace and strength here that we couldn't have imagined. Thank you for bringing this sanctuary to Kenya."

As the foundation's global network grew, Chrissy and her team continued to innovate and expand their support programs. They launched virtual support groups and telemedicine services, allowing families who couldn't travel to the hospices to still receive care and connect with others facing similar challenges.

One evening, back at the Caribbean hospice, Chrissy reflected on the incredible journey they had undertaken. The foundation's network now spanned five continents, each hospice serving as a beacon of hope and support for families affected by PSP.

Chrissy received a call from Dr. Aisha Malik, the researcher whose groundbreaking work on gene therapy had shown significant promise.

"Chrissy, I have exciting news," Dr. Malik said. "Our clinical trials have yielded remarkable results. We're seeing significant improvements in patients' motor functions and quality of life. I believe we're on the verge of a major breakthrough."

Chrissy's heart swelled with hope. "That's incredible, Dr. Malik. Your work is changing lives, and I can't wait to see where this leads. Let's plan to expand these trials to our hospices worldwide."

With renewed determination, the foundation began to roll out the new gene therapy trials at their global hospices. Families who had once felt hopeless now had access to cutting-edge treatments, giving them a renewed sense of hope and possibility.

The foundation's efforts continued to gain international recognition. Chrissy was invited to speak at global health conferences, sharing the foundation's mission and the incredible progress they had made. Her speeches inspired other organizations and individuals to join the fight against PSP, creating a ripple effect of support and innovation.

One day, as Chrissy walked through the gardens of the original Caribbean hospice, she felt a profound sense of fulfillment. The foundation had grown beyond her wildest dreams, driven by the love and resilience of countless families and supporters.

She knew that the journey was far from over. There were still many families who needed their help, many lives to touch, and many memories to create. But she felt confident that with the foundation's unwavering commitment and the enduring spirit of her mother, Sara, they could continue to make a difference.

As the sun set over the tranquil waters, Chrissy made a silent vow to keep pushing forward, to keep expanding their horizons, and to keep bringing hope and healing to families around the world. The Sara Jones Foundation had become a global force for good, and its mission to honor Sara's legacy and support families affected by PSP would continue to inspire and transform lives for generations to come.

Chapter 13: The Path to a Cure

The Sara Jones Foundation had reached incredible heights, transforming the lives of families affected by PSP across the globe. With their network of respite hospices, innovative research, and unwavering support, they had become a beacon of hope. Yet, Chrissy knew their ultimate goal was to find a cure for PSP, and they were closer than ever before.

One morning, Chrissy received an urgent call from Dr. Elena Rossi. The excitement in Dr. Rossi's voice was palpable.

"Chrissy, I have groundbreaking news," Dr. Rossi said. "Our latest research has identified a potential cure for PSP. The gene therapy trials have shown remarkable results, and we're ready to move to the next phase."

Chrissy's heart raced with hope. "That's incredible, Dr. Rossi. What do we need to do to bring this cure to families around the world?"

Dr. Rossi explained that they needed to conduct large-scale clinical trials to confirm the therapy's effectiveness and ensure it met regulatory standards. This would require significant funding and collaboration with medical institutions worldwide.

Chrissy immediately called a board meeting, sharing the exhilarating news with her team. They agreed to launch a massive fundraising campaign, aiming to secure the resources needed to bring the potential cure to market.

The campaign, named "Path to a Cure," kicked off with a global event, featuring live-streamed speeches, musical performances, and testimonials from families who had benefited from the foundation's work. Chrissy's speech was a highlight of the event.

"Today, we stand on the brink of a medical breakthrough," Chrissy announced to the global audience. "The Sara Jones Foundation has always been driven by the hope and resilience of families affected by PSP. With your support, we can bring this potential cure to those who need it most. Together, we can make history."

The response was overwhelming. Donations poured in from individuals, corporations, and philanthropic organizations worldwide. Celebrities and influencers joined the cause, using their platforms to raise awareness and funds. Within weeks, the foundation had secured the necessary resources to move forward with the clinical trials.

Dr. Rossi and her team began coordinating with medical institutions in each region where the foundation had a hospice. The trials would be conducted at these sites, ensuring that families had access to the latest treatments and support during the process.

Chrissy traveled to each hospice, meeting with researchers, healthcare providers, and families. She shared updates on the trials and reassured everyone that they were on the cusp of something truly transformative.

One evening, while visiting the hospice in Tuscany, Chrissy sat with Maria, one of the trial participants, and her family.

"Chrissy, this gene therapy has given us hope we never thought possible," Maria said, holding Chrissy's hand. "Thank you for fighting for us."

Chrissy felt a surge of emotion. "Maria, your strength and courage inspire us every day. We're in this together, and we won't stop until we find a cure."

As the trials progressed, the results continued to be promising. Patients showed significant improvements in their symptoms, and the data confirmed the therapy's potential to halt and even reverse the progression of PSP. The foundation's researchers worked tirelessly, analyzing the data and preparing for the next steps.

Months later, Dr. Rossi called Chrissy with the news they had all been waiting for.

"Chrissy, the trials have been a success," Dr. Rossi said, her voice filled with joy. "We've submitted our findings to the regulatory authorities, and I'm confident we'll receive approval soon. This is it – we've found a cure for PSP."

Tears filled Chrissy's eyes as she shared the news with her team and the families at the hospices. Celebrations erupted across the foundation's global network. It was a moment of triumph, the culmination of years of hard work, dedication, and unwavering hope.

The regulatory approval came swiftly, and the gene therapy was made available to patients worldwide. The foundation's hospices became centers for administering the treatment, ensuring that families received the best care and support during the process.

The impact was immediate and profound. Families who had once faced a bleak future now had hope. Patients regained their abilities, their lives transformed by the therapy. The foundation's mission had come full circle, from providing respite and support to delivering a cure.

She felt her mother's presence, guiding her every step of the way. Sara's legacy had inspired a global movement, one that had changed the course of PSP and brought hope to countless lives.

As the sun set over the tranquil waters, Chrissy made a silent vow to continue their work, to keep pushing forward, and to bring hope and healing to families around the world. The Sara Jones Foundation had become a global force for good, and its mission to honor Sara's legacy and support families affected by PSP would continue to inspire and transform lives for generations to come.

Through the triumphs and challenges, the foundation's spirit remained unbreakable. Together, they had forged a path to a cure, and their journey was a testament to the power of love, determination, and the enduring legacy of an extraordinary woman.

Chapter 14: A Lasting Legacy

With the monumental achievement of finding a cure for PSP, the Sara Jones Foundation had reached a new pinnacle. The world was now aware of their incredible journey and their relentless pursuit of a cure. However, Chrissy knew that their mission was far from over. There were still many challenges to face and countless families who needed their help.

One day, Chrissy received a call from David, the tech entrepreneur who had been instrumental in modernizing the foundation's digital presence.

"Chrissy, we've done something extraordinary, but we need to think about the future," David said. "How can we ensure that the foundation's work continues to grow and impact more lives?"

Chrissy agreed wholeheartedly. "You're right, David. We need to build on our success and continue to innovate. Let's start by expanding our scope to include other neurodegenerative diseases and ensure our support systems remain strong."

The foundation began to focus on expanding their research efforts and forming new partnerships. They aimed to include more neurodegenerative diseases such as Alzheimer's, Parkinson's, and ALS in their scope. The foundation's respite hospices became centers of excellence for neurodegenerative disease research and care, offering hope to even more families.

One day, while visiting the hospice in Tuscany, Chrissy met with Dr. Luca Marino, a renowned researcher in Alzheimer's disease.

"Dr. Marino, we're excited to collaborate with you," Chrissy said. "Our experience with PSP has shown us the power of innovative research and comprehensive care. Together, we can make a difference for families affected by Alzheimer's."

Dr. Marino smiled warmly. "Chrissy, your foundation's work is truly inspiring. I'm honored to join forces with you and bring hope to those facing the challenges of Alzheimer's."

The collaboration led to the development of new therapies and support programs, further solidifying the foundation's reputation as a leader in neurological research and care.

As the foundation continued to grow and evolve, Chrissy remained committed to their core mission. She traveled frequently, visiting each hospice, meeting with researchers, and ensuring that every family received the highest standard of care and support.

The foundation's impact extended beyond the families they directly served. Their research and advocacy efforts influenced healthcare policies and funding, raising awareness about neurodegenerative diseases and the importance of comprehensive care.

Moving Forward

The story of Chrissy and the Sara Jones Foundation is a testament to the incredible impact one person can make when driven by love, hope, and determination. While the characters and events in this book are fictional, the spirit of their journey is very real and resonates deeply with the experiences of countless families affected by neurodegenerative diseases.

As you close this book, I hope you feel inspired by Chrissy's unwavering commitment to her mother's legacy and the difference she made in the lives of so many. The challenges faced by those with neurodegenerative diseases are profound, but so too is the potential for each of us to contribute to the fight against these conditions.

I urge you to be the Chrissy in your community. Whether it's through supporting a loved one, volunteering your time, advocating for better healthcare policies, or contributing to research efforts, every action counts. You have the power to bring hope, support, and change to those who need it most.

Together, we can build a world where neurodegenerative diseases are met not with despair but with hope and resilience. We can honor the legacies of those we've lost by continuing their fight and striving for a future where every family has access to the care and support they need.

Thank you for joining me on this journey. Now, let us take the next steps together, inspired by Chrissy's story, and make a lasting difference in the world.

About the Author: Laura Louizos

54

Laura Louizos is a compassionate advocate and caregiver who founded the Coleen Cunningham Foundation in honor of her mother, Coleen Cunningham, who bravely battled Progressive Supranuclear Palsy (PSP). Throughout her mother's journey, Laura was her primary caregiver, experiencing firsthand the challenges and triumphs that come with caring for a loved one with a neurodegenerative disease.

Inspired by her mother's strength and resilience, Laura dedicated herself to supporting families and individuals affected by PSP. The Coleen Cunningham Foundation focuses on providing comprehensive support, respite care, and resources to help families navigate the complexities of living with PSP. Laura's work is centered on ensuring that no family faces this journey alone, offering emotional and practical support at every step.

No One Walks Alone
For resources and support visit:
pspawareness.com